Healing Hearts

How to Protect and Improve Your Heart Health

Jessica Hensley.

Table of contents

Chapter 1
Chapter 2
Chapter 3

Chapter 1

Knowing cardiovascular illness

Problems with the heart and blood arteries are often referred to as cardiovascular disease. Atherosclerosis is frequently the cause of these issues. When cholesterol and fat deposit in the walls of arteries, a disease known as atherosclerosis results. The accumulation is known as plaque. Plaque can constrict blood arteries over time, leading to issues throughout the body. A heart attack or stroke may result from a clogged artery.

Cardiovascular Disease Types

The most prevalent kind of heart illness, coronary heart disease (CHD), occurs when plaque accumulates in the arteries that supply the heart. An alternative name for CHD is coronary artery disease (CAD). The heart cannot get enough blood and oxygen when arteries are constricted. A heart attack may result from an arterial blockage. Heart failure or arrhythmias can develop over time as a result of CHD weakening the heart muscle.

When the heart muscle becomes rigid or weak, cardiac failure ensues. The body has symptoms because it cannot pump enough oxygen-rich blood. Only the right or only the left side of the heart may be impacted by the illness. Both halves of the heart are more frequently implicated. Heart failure is frequently brought on by CAD and high blood pressure.

Problems with cardiac rhythm or pace are referred to as arrhythmias. When the heart's electrical system is malfunctioning, this occurs. The heart's rhythm may be irregular, excessively rapid, or too sluggish. The electrical system of the heart can become faulty as a result of several cardiac conditions, such as heart attack or heart failure. Some individuals are born with an arrhythmia.

When one of the heart's four valves is malfunctioning, heart valve disorders might develop. Regurgitation is the term for when blood leaks through a valve in the incorrect direction, and stenosis is the term for when a valve does not open all the way. The most typical sign is a heart murmur, which is an abnormal heartbeat. Heart valve disorders can be brought on by specific heart issues such as heart attacks, heart illness, or infections. Some people have heart valve issues from birth.

The arteries leading to your legs and feet constrict as a result of a buildup of plaque, which is referred to as peripheral arterial disease. Blood flow is impeded or reduced by narrow arteries. Nerves and tissue might get damaged when the legs are deprived of blood and oxygen.

Heart attack, heart failure, and stroke are just a few of the complications that can result from high blood pressure (also known as hypertension), a cardiovascular illness.

Strokes are brought on by inadequate blood supply to the brain. This may occur as a result of bleeding inside the brain or a blood clot moving to the blood arteries there. Heart disease and stroke have many of the same risk factors.

A structural or functional issue with the heart that exists from birth is referred to as congenital heart disease. Many distinct cardiac conditions can be categorized as congenital heart disease. The most typical kind of birth defect is this one.

Why do cardiovascular diseases occur?

Depending on the exact form, cardiovascular disease can have a variety of causes. For instance, coronary artery disease and peripheral artery disease are brought on by atherosclerosis (plaque accumulation in your arteries). Arrhythmias can be brought on by coronary artery disease, cardiac muscle scarring, hereditary issues, or drug side effects. Valve problems can be brought on by aging, infections, and rheumatic illness.

What are the risk factors for cardiovascular disease? If you have risk factors like these, you might be more prone to develop cardiovascular disease:

• High blood pressure (hypertension).
• High cholesterol (hyperlipidemia).
• Tobacco use (including vaping).
• Type 2 diabetes.
• Family history of heart disease.
• Lack of physical activity.
• Having excess weight or obesity.
• Diet high in sodium, sugar and fat.
• Overuse of alcohol.
• Misuse of prescription or recreational drugs.
• Preeclampsia or toxemia.
• Gestational diabetes.

• Chronic inflammatory or autoimmune conditions.
• Chronic kidney disease.

Diabetes increases your chance of developing heart disease. This condition, which is also known as cardiovascular disease (CVD) or coronary disease, can cause strokes and heart attacks.

Your circulation is also impacted by cardiovascular disease. Additionally, additional diabetic consequences, such as issues with your eyes and feet, are made worse by poor circulation.
Because of this, it's critical to look after your heart while you have diabetes. We're here to explain why having diabetes raises your chance of developing heart issues and how to lower that risk.

Why does diabetes make you more likely to get heart disease?

Even modestly elevated blood sugar levels over time can cause damage to your blood vessels, which can result in significant cardiac problems.

This is because your body can't adequately utilize all of this sugar, which causes more of it to adhere to your red blood cells and accumulate in your blood. The blood veins delivering blood to and from your heart may get blocked and damaged as a result of this buildup, depriving the heart of oxygen and nutrients.

Therefore, maintaining your HbA1c level as near to your goal as feasible can assist to safeguard your blood vessels and, in turn, your heart. Over time, even slightly elevated blood sugar levels can.

High triglycerides
The additional fat in your blood adheres to the walls of your blood vessels if your cholesterol level is too high. This fat becomes hard over time and is referred to as plaque.
The blood arteries may get blocked by hard plaque, which will make the passageway smaller and less conducive to blood flow. The most frequent reason for a heart attack is a condition known as atherosclerosis or arteriosclerosis.

Blood flow slows down in the smaller area, which leads to certain blood cells congregating and clotting. If a blood clot separates, it will move through your veins and arteries until it encounters a passageway that is too narrow for it to pass through, blocking it partially or entirely.

By depriving the heart of oxygen and nourishment, this can result in a heart attack.

High blood pressure
Not only does the blood struggle to pass through the blood vessels, but as time passes, atherosclerosis causes the blood vessel walls to become less flexible and more hard. This can either cause or exacerbate high blood pressure, often known as hypertension.

Your blood vessels are also put under additional strain by high blood pressure. On top of the stress caused by excessive cholesterol and blood sugar, that is.

Blood vessel narrowing might also affect other body parts, such as your legs and feet. Peripheral vascular disease (PVD) is what it is known as, and if ignored, it can result in amputation. By taking care of yourself, you can lessen the risk of blood vessel deterioration.

• blood sugar levels
• blood pressure
• cholesterol (blood fats)

If you have diabetes, you should have regular checkups that include having your cholesterol, blood pressure, and HbA1c measured. You should be able to receive your diabetic healthcare checks as usual, but if you continue to encounter cancellations or delays due to the coronavirus pandemic, we urge that you contact your healthcare team to find out when these issues will arise once again.

You can control your diabetes and guard yourself against heart problems by keeping an eye on these three things. But you may take a variety of additional steps to lower your chance of developing heart disease.
lowering your risk of heart disease or a heart attack
The good news is that you can lower your chance of getting heart disease or having a heart attack.

This is how:

• As part of your annual diabetes review, have your HbA1c, blood pressure, and blood cholesterol (blood fats) checked at least once a year. Be sure to obtain guidance and assistance from your healthcare team to keep these measurements within your goal range.

• Seek aid to quit smoking. Blood flow is hampered by smoking, especially when it comes to the heart. Ask your healthcare staff for extra assistance if you need it, or go over our material to assist you with quitting.

• Maintain a heart-healthy, well-balanced diet.

• Exercise often and keep yourself physically active.

• If you need assistance losing weight, seek it out if you are obese or overweight. A modest loss can have a significant impact.

· Follow the directions on your prescriptions. Even if you don't have blood pressure issues or excessive blood fat levels, you can still take several medications that protect your heart by lowering these conditions.

Chapter 2

signs of a heart attack in women

The most typical heart attack symptom in women is the same as in men: a persistent or intermittent form of chest pain, pressure, or discomfort.

However, especially in women, chest discomfort is not usually severe or even the most obvious sign. Pressure or tightness is a common way for women to describe heart attack pain. Additionally, a heart attack can occur without chest discomfort.

In contrast to males, women are more prone to experience heart attack symptoms like:

• Neck, jaw, shoulder, upper back or upper belly (abdomen) discomfort
• Shortness of breath
• Pain in one or both arms
• Nausea or vomiting
• Sweating
• Lightheadedness or dizziness

- Unusual fatigue
- Heartburn (indigestion)

These signs and symptoms might not be as obvious as the severe chest discomfort that is frequently connected to heart attacks. This may be due to small vessel heart disease, also known as coronary microvascular disease, a condition in which women are more likely than males to have blockages not just in their major arteries but also in the smaller ones that feed blood to the heart.

Women typically experience sensations more frequently than men do when relaxing or even asleep. In women, emotional stress may contribute to the onset of heart attack symptoms.

Women may experience fewer heart disease diagnoses than males since women's heart attack symptoms might be different from men's. Without a major arterial blockage, women are more likely than men to get a heart attack.

Women's heart disease risk factors

Women and men are both affected by a number of the classic risk factors for coronary artery disease, including excessive cholesterol, high blood pressure, and obesity. However, other variables may contribute more to the onset of heart disease in women.

Risk factors for heart disease in women include:

• Diabetology. Compared to males with diabetes, women have a higher risk of developing heart disease. There is also a higher chance of experiencing a silent heart attack, which has no visible signs, as diabetes can alter how painful things feel for women.

• Depression and emotional stress. Women's hearts are more susceptible to stress and depression than men's. Maintaining a healthy lifestyle and adhering to treatment recommendations for various medical disorders may be challenging for someone who is depressed.

• Cigarettes. Compared to males, women are more at risk for heart disease from smoking.

• The menopause. Following menopause, low estrogen levels raise the risk of illness in smaller blood arteries.

• Problems related to pregnancy. Diabetes or high blood pressure during pregnancy can raise the mother's long-term chance of developing these conditions. Women are likewise more prone to get heart disease due to these problems.

• A history of early heart disease in the family. This seems to be a risk factor that affects women more than males.

• Diseases with inflammation. Both men and women may have an increased risk of developing heart disease as a result of rheumatoid arthritis, lupus, and other inflammatory diseases.

Heart disease should be taken seriously by women of all ages. Heart disease risk factors are particularly important for women under the age of 65 who have a family history of the condition. A healthy lifestyle can lower the chance of developing heart disease. Try the following heart-healthy techniques:

• Give up smoking. Stop smoking if you don't already. Avoid secondhand smoke as much as you can because it can potentially harm your blood vessels.

• Consume a balanced diet. Choose lean meats, whole grains, fruits, and vegetables as well as low-fat or fat-free dairy products. Steer clear of additional sweets, saturated or trans fats, and a lot of salt.

• Maintain a healthy weight through exercise. Even a small weight loss can reduce your chance of developing heart disease if you are overweight. Find out what weight is ideal for you by speaking with your doctor.
Some techniques for managing stress include increasing physical activity, engaging in mindfulness exercises, and forming supportive relationships.

• Limit alcohol consumption. If you decide to consume alcohol, do so sparingly. That entails up to one drink per day for women and up to two drinks per day for males for healthy individuals.

· Adhere to your treatment schedule. Aspirin, blood thinners, and other prescription drugs should be taken exactly as directed.

• Take care of other medical issues. Diabetes, high cholesterol, and high blood pressure all raise the risk of developing heart disease.

Heart health and exercise
The heart is kept healthy by regular exercise. On most days of the week, try to get in at least 30 minutes of moderate activity, such as brisk walking. Start small and work your way up if that's more than you can handle. Exercising for even five minutes a day is good for your health.

Aim for 60 minutes of moderate to intense activity each day, five days a week, for greater health improvement. Additionally, perform weight training activities twice a week or more.

It's acceptable to divide your workouts into many 10-minute intervals throughout the day. The advantages for your heart's health remain the same.

Another strategy to sustain a healthy weight, lower blood pressure, and maintain heart health is through interval training, which alternates brief bursts of intensive exercise with intervals of moderate activity. For instance, incorporate brief bursts of running or quick walking with your daily strolls.

With this advice, you may include fitness into your everyday routine:

• Take the stairs instead of an elevator.
• Walk or ride your bike to work or to do errands.
• March in place while watching television.

Treatment for heart disease in women

Treatment for heart disease is generally the same for men and women. Medication, angioplasty and stenting procedures, or cardiac bypass surgery are all possible.

Men and women are treated differently for heart disease, with several distinctions being noted:

• Compared to males, women are less likely to receive aspirin and statin therapy to stave off further heart attacks. Studies indicate that both groups receive comparable advantages, nevertheless.

• Women are less likely than males to undergo coronary bypass surgery, maybe because they have smaller arteries or less obstructive disease in their arteries.

• Cardiac rehab can boost well-being and speed up recovery from heart illness. However, compared to males, women are less frequently recommended for cardiac rehabilitation.

Your body uses cholesterol to generate hormones, insulate neurons, and create new cells. The liver typically produces all the cholesterol the body requires. But dietary sources of cholesterol also include items derived from animals, such as milk, eggs, and meat. Cardiovascular disease is a risk factor for having too much cholesterol in your body.

How Does Heart Disease Relate to High Cholesterol?

Atherosclerosis, a kind of heart disease, is a process that occurs when there is an excessive buildup of cholesterol in the artery walls. Blood flow to the heart muscle is reduced or restricted when the arteries constrict.

If not enough blood and oxygen reach your heart, you may have chest discomfort. Blood transports oxygen to the heart. A heart attack occurs when a blockage entirely cuts off the blood flow to a section of the heart.

Most people are aware of the following two types of cholesterol: LDL, or "bad" cholesterol, and HDL, or "good" cholesterol, are two types of lipoproteins. These are the ways that cholesterol manifests itself in the blood.

Plaque that clogs arteries is mostly produced by LDL. In reality, HDL helps to remove cholesterol from the blood.

Triglycerides are another kind of fat found in our blood. Recent studies suggest that triglyceride levels over normal may potentially be associated with heart disease.

What Are High Cholesterol Symptoms?

Since high cholesterol does not in and of itself manifest any symptoms, many people are unaware that they have elevated cholesterol. As a result, it's critical to learn your cholesterol levels. Too-high cholesterol levels increase the risk of acquiring heart disease and, if you already have it, increase the likelihood of having a heart attack or passing away from the condition.

Regarding Heart Health, High Blood Pressure Management

1. Exercise regularly
According to ResearchTrusted Source, both aerobic and strength training can help prevent or control high blood pressure, and the hours following a workout may see a reduction in blood pressure.

Tips for increasing your activity levels include:

• using the stairs
• walking instead of driving
• doing household chores
• gardening
• going for a bike ride
• playing a team sport

2. Control weight

The heart and cardiovascular system are strained when a person is carrying around extra body weight. This could make blood pressure go up.

Losing 5–10 pounds can help lower your blood pressure if your body mass index (BMI) is 25 or above. It may also reduce the likelihood of developing other health issues.

The three most effective strategies to do this are to:

• Eat less.
• Eat well.

3. Consume less refined carbs and sugars

Limiting sugar and processed carbs may aid in weight loss and blood pressure reduction.

Low-carb, low-fat diets reduced systolic and diastolic blood pressure in overweight or obese people by an average of 3 mm Hg and nearly 5 mm Hg, respectively.

4. Less salt and more potassium

Salt consumption needs to be reduced, along with potassium intake, to lower blood pressure.

High salt consumption can raise the risk. Reducing salt intake decreases blood pressure, according to a reliable source. Although the specific cause is unknown to experts, water retention and blood vessel inflammation may play a role. Potassium reduces blood vessel stress and aids in the body's process of eliminating salt.

foods high in potassium include:

• dried fruit like prunes and apricots
• Yogurt and milk
• kidney beans and lentils
• veggies like spinach, tomatoes, and potatoes

5. Consuming a heart-healthy diet
The DASH (Dietary Approaches to Stop Hypertension) programme is suggested by the National Institutes of Health as a heart-healthy alternative.

The DASH diet focuses on:

• consuming whole grains, veggies, and fruits
• eating dairy products with little or no fat.

• consuming vegetable oils, beans, nuts, fish, and poultry
• avoiding meals high in added sugars and saturated fats

6. Avoid processed foods.
Processed foods frequently include excessive levels of salt, sugar, and bad fats. They could make you put on weight. All of these things can raise blood pressure. Examples comprise:

• Finished meats
• a lot of fried or quick food
• Prepared foods

Low-fat foods may contain a lot of salt and sugar to make up for the lost fat. Food tastes better and makes you feel full when it is fatty.
You may reduce your intake of refined carbs, salt, and sugar by eating less processed foods. Lower blood pressure can be the outcome of all of these.

7. Give up or don't smoke
Your whole health, including your blood pressure, might be impacted by smoking.

The compounds in cigarettes can raise your blood pressure over time by:

• causing damage to the blood vessel walls
• triggering swelling
• making your arteries smaller.
Higher blood pressure is a result of the hardened arteries.
Even when exposed to secondhand smoke, the compounds in tobacco can harm your blood vessels.

8. Stress Control
Your health and blood pressure depend on you learning how to manage stress.
Depending on the person, there are a variety of ways to reduce stress, such as:

• using deep breathing exercises
• going for a walk
• reading book
• listening to music
• Awareness
• mindfulness

9. Consume some chocolate.

Cacao content ranges between 70 and 85% in dark chocolate.

Flavonoids, an antioxidant found in cacao, may help decrease blood pressure. Your blood arteries may dilate or expand with the aid of these flavonoids. The American Heart Association points out that while consuming a little quantity of dark chocolate is unlikely to be dangerous, doing so daily is unlikely to offer enough flavonoids to have a positive impact on health.

High sugar, fat, or calorie chocolate could not be healthy.

10. Examine these healing plants.

Certain herbal remedies may assist in lowering blood pressure. To determine the dosages and elements in the herbs that are most effective, additional study is necessary.

Several herbs and plants are used by individuals to decrease blood pressure including:

• black bean (*Castanospermum australe*)
• cat's claw (*Uncaria rhynchophylla*)
• celery juice (*Apium graveolens*)
• Chinese hawthorn (*Crataegus pinnatifida*)
• ginger root

• giant dodder (*Cuscuta reflexa*)
• Indian plantago (blond psyllium)
• maritime pine bark (*Pinus pinaster*)
• river lily (*Crinum glaucum*)
• Roselle (*Hibiscus sabdariffa*)
• sesame oil (*Sesamum indicum*)
• tomato extract (*Lycopersicon esculentum*)
• tea (*Camellia sinensis*), especially green tea and oolong tea

11. Get sufficient rest.
Lack of sleep may make people more susceptible to high blood pressure.
Your blood pressure normally drops as you sleep, which might be one of the causes. If you have trouble sleeping, you might not go through this phase.
The following are suggestions for getting a good night's sleep:

• establishing a consistent sleep routine
• working out during the day, but not just before bed
• slumbering in a cool, dark space
• using electronic devices outside of the bedroom
• avoiding eating, drinking, or using caffeine or alcohol too soon before night

Obtain advice on how to sleep soundly.

12. Consume garlic or supplement with garlic extract
Foods high in protein include

• fish, such as salmon or canned tuna in water
• eggs
• poultry, such as chicken breast
• lean beef
• beans and legumes, such as kidney beans and lentils
• nuts or nut butter, such as peanut butter
• chickpeas
•low-fat cheese and other dairy products

A doctor should be consulted before changing to a high-protein diet because not everyone should do so. Additionally, it's critical to strike a balance between various protein sources and other nutrients.

13. Reduce blood pressure by taking vitamins.
14. Consume wholesome, high-protein meals
15. Add vitamins to your diet to reduce blood pressure
A beverage is

*Four ounces of wine
*one 12-ounce beer
*1.5 ounces of alcohol at 80 proof
* A single ounce of 100-proof alcohol

Examine your caffeine consumption
Those who typically drink 1-3 cups of coffee a day are unlikely to see their blood pressure go up.
However, if you drink a lot of coffee—or even a little—when you're not used to it, your blood pressure can increase.
On the other hand, energy drinks containing a lot of caffeine may raise blood pressure and, thus, the risk of cardiovascular issues. Energy drink intake is not recommended by experts, especially for young people with pre-existing medical concerns. Try decaffeinated coffee if you notice that caffeine is making you feel unwell.

17. Sip some water
In addition to its many other potential advantages, water can improve general health.

18. Use prescription drugs

Depending on your blood pressure level and other variables, your doctor may advise taking prescription medicines from Trusted Source if your blood pressure is high or doesn't drop after making these lifestyle modifications.

Chapter 3

How common is CVD worldwide?

One of the largest hazards to human health today is cardiovascular disease (CVD), which is a major worry for worldwide medical and scientific communities. Currently, cardiovascular diseases (CVDs) such as coronary heart disease (CHD) and stroke account for 31% of all fatalities worldwide, killing an estimated 17.5 million people annually1. In the US, it is the leading cause of death for both sexes2, and one in five individuals in China is thought to have it, with the nation having one of the highest CVD mortality rates in the world3.

Which are the primary causes of CVD risk?

There are two types of risk factors: those that cannot be changed, like age, and those that can. Surprisingly many of the latter may be traced to lifestyle choices, including smoking, having high blood pressure, having raised blood lipid levels, living a sedentary lifestyle, being obese, and, most crucially, eating poorly. Blood pressure, blood lipids, and the prevalence of a sedentary lifestyle can all be improved by bringing one's body mass index (BMI) down to the "normal" range of 20 to 25 kg/m2. If BMI is already within this range, this can be done by keeping calorie intake the same, or by maintaining a negative calorie balance while increasing activity to burn more calories if BMI is higher than 25 kg/m.

Changing one's lifestyle can sometimes be difficult, impractical, or takes time, although many risk factors are tied to it. In such circumstances, medications are required to address raised blood lipid levels, and additional medications can be used to manage high blood pressure or even smoking addiction.

One's diet composition is a significant contributor to the development of CVD. The Western diet, which is becoming more and more popular across the world, is low in whole grains, nuts and seeds, vitamin D, and marine-based omega-3 fatty acids (EPA and DHA). It is also high in salt and sugar-sweetened drinks. As a result, those who follow this diet are more likely to get a heart attack, stroke, type 2 diabetes, or possibly pass away. As a result, those who follow this diet are more likely to get heart attacks, strokes, type 2 diabetes, and even pass away, with dietary variables thought to be responsible for a sizable share of fatalities. In contrast, it has been shown that the Mediterranean diet, which is high in nuts, oily fish, fruits, and vegetables and low in red meat, salt, and sugar-sweetened drinks, lowers the risk of cardiovascular events.

Additionally, there is a significant association between several biomarkers, such as diabetes, and CVD. According to the American Heart Association, persons with diabetes have a four times higher risk of dying from heart disease than adults without the illness.
Recommendations for lowering the risk of CVD through contributing lifestyle variables.

Regional recommendations differ, but it is generally accepted that those with a high risk of CVD should consume a diet rich in fruits, vegetables, whole grains, lean meats, poultry, fish, nuts, legumes, and seeds with less added sugar. As people are not always following current guidance, it is challenging to rely on patients to make adjustments to dramatically improve their lifestyles. This is partially caused by patients' and even doctors' lack of understanding of what makes up a well-balanced, healthy diet and how to attain it. The supply of vital elements in an individual has recently been measured using biomarkers. The most sophisticated biomarkers are for vitamin D and omega-3 fatty acids (EPA; DHA), and it has been discovered that a significant fraction of the people studied is deficient in these two nutrients. As new research becomes available, guidelines are always changing.

What part does diet play in promoting heart health?

A balanced, nutrient-rich diet can assist to avoid or significantly lower the risk of developing CVD, just as poor nutrition can play a significant role in raising the risk. According to the World Health Organization (WHO), lifestyle modifications can prevent 75 percent of CVD-related deaths, and there is mounting evidence that certain diets and minerals can have an impact on CVD risk. Numerous studies have also shown that essential minerals, such as vitamin D and the omega-3 fatty acids eicosapentaenoic acid (EPA) and docosahexaenoic acid (DHA), can promote heart health.

What proof exists that EPA and DHA from the omega-3 family reduce the risk factors for cardiovascular disease?

Omega-3 EPA and DHA may assist to lower the risk of developing CVD, according to mounting data. Furthermore, EPA and DHA supplementation significantly decreased the risk of CHD in those with increased triglycerides or LDL cholesterol, according to a recent meta-analysis of studies investigating the link between EPA and DHA on CHD. However, a sizable portion of big interventional studies using EPA and DHA supplementation in cardiovascular disease revealed either negative or neutral findings. The use of EPA and DHA supplements in the recommendations for cardiovascular prevention is thus not currently supported by the European Society of Cardiology (ESC). It is unlikely that the limited positive or neutral results of these experiments may be attributed to EPA and DHA's inefficiency. By assessing EPA and DHA levels using the standardized HS-Omega-3 Index®, it was recently discovered that the issue is more with the bioavailability of EPA and DHA and problems with the trial methodology. A new generation of level-based major intervention trials, according to many, is now required to better depict and comprehend how EPA and DHA affect cardiovascular health.

However, the American Heart Association (AHA) recently released a statement strongly endorsing the use of EPA and DHA supplements in congestive heart failure and, less strongly, in patients who have recently suffered a heart attack, based on encouraging results from some trials and the entirety of the evidence.

What proof is there that vitamin D helps prevent CVD from killing people off?

Higher levels of vitamin D have been linked to lifespan and a decrease in the occurrence of cardiovascular events in addition to its traditional role in preserving bone health.
When vitamin D levels fall below 30 ng/ml, equal to 25(OH) vitamin D levels in serum, the risk of death and cardiovascular events rises.

Managing high blood pressure and lowering the risk of hypertension and CHD are two additional benefits of vitamin D. Cardiovascular organizations do not now advocate the use of vitamin D as a supplement, although a meta-analysis of intervention studies indicated that increasing consumption of the vitamin decreases overall mortality, even if a daily dose of up to 100 g is deemed safe by the EFSA. Adults can safely consume up to 100 mg, or 4000 I.E., of vitamin D3 per day to reach optimal vitamin D levels.

What about other vital nutrients?
Important nutrients, such as vitamins C and E, as well as soluble fibers like oat beta-glucan, have also been discovered to enhance heart function.

Vitamin E is known to help protect cells from harm and preserve arterial health. It has also been associated with a decreased risk of cardiovascular disease owing to oxidative stress and inflammation. Vitamin C, on the other hand, has been shown to help heart health; higher levels of the vitamin have been associated with lower blood pressure and better vasodilation in those with CHD.
Oat beta-glucan's ability to decrease cholesterol and, as a result, the risk of developing heart disease, has been emphasized by research on soluble fibers. In

the EU, oat beta-glucan for daily consumption of 3 g has been allowed in 2011 with a claim on the reduction of a disease risk factor: It has been demonstrated that oat beta-glucan lowers or reduces blood cholesterol. A risk factor for the onset of coronary heart disease is high cholesterol.

• Physical Activity and Exercise for a Healthy Heart

Physical activity is one of the finest gifts you can offer your heart. A healthy lifestyle that includes regular exercise, a Mediterranean-style diet, keeping a normal weight, and quitting smoking offers the best defense against coronary artery disease and vascular disease.

• hinder the progression of diabetes.
Regular aerobic exercise, such as cycling, brisk walking, or swimming, can lower the risk of developing diabetes by over 50% when combined with strength training. This is because it improves the muscles' ability to process glycogen, a fuel for energy that, when impaired, results in high blood sugar levels and diabetes.

• Stress is reduced through exercise.

The heart may be further burdened by stress chemicals. Exercise may help you unwind and reduce stress, whether it is aerobic (like jogging), resistance-focused (like weight training), or flexibility-focused (like yoga).

• Inflammation is reduced by exercise.
As the body adjusts to the demands of exercise on several physical systems, chronic inflammation is lessened with regular exercise. This is crucial for minimizing the negative impacts of many of the disorders we just discussed.